Chapter 1: Understanding Early Onset Dementia

Defining Early Onset Dementia

Early onset dementia refers to a form of dementia that occurs in individuals under the age of 65. While dementia is often associated with older adults, early onset dementia presents unique challenges, both for patients and their caregivers. This condition encompasses various types, including Alzheimer's disease, frontotemporal dementia, and other neurodegenerative disorders. Understanding the specific characteristics and symptoms of early onset dementia is critical for effective management and support, as the experiences and needs of younger individuals diagnosed with this condition can differ significantly from those of older patients.

Symptoms of early onset dementia can be subtle and may initially resemble typical age-related changes. Common indicators include memory loss, difficulty with problem-solving or planning, challenges in language and communication, and changes in mood or personality. Unlike typical dementia, which may progress gradually, early onset dementia can have a more rapid progression, leading to significant impairments in daily functioning. It is essential for patients and their families to recognize these symptoms early, as timely diagnosis and intervention can provide opportunities for better management and quality of life.

The diagnosis of early onset dementia often involves a comprehensive evaluation by healthcare professionals, including neurologists and geriatric specialists. This process may include cognitive assessments, brain imaging, and laboratory tests to rule out other conditions. Given the age of onset, patients may face additional complexities, such as navigating employment challenges, family dynamics, and financial planning. Engaging with a multisciplinary team can provide valuable resources and support tailored to the unique needs of younger individuals facing dementia.

Living with early onset dementia requires a proactive approach to care and engagement. Patients and caregivers can benefit from incorporating dementia-friendly activities into their daily routines, promoting cognitive stimulation and social interaction. These activities can range from memory games to art projects, allowing individuals to connect with others while maintaining a sense of purpose. Additionally, focusing on nutrition and diet can play a significant role in overall health and may even contribute to the management of cognitive decline. A balanced diet, rich in antioxidants and omega-3 fatty acids, is often recommended.

Legal and financial planning becomes increasingly important for individuals diagnosed with early onset dementia, as they may still have significant responsibilities and commitments. Establishing advance directives, power of attorney, and exploring long-term care options can alleviate future stress for both patients and their families. Furthermore, staying informed about ongoing dementia research and clinical trials can provide insights into potential treatments and innovations in care. By fostering open communication strategies and seeking support from caregiver networks, individuals living with early onset dementia can navigate their journey with greater confidence and resilience.

Symptoms and Diagnosis

Symptoms of early onset dementia can vary significantly from person to person, but common indicators often include memory loss, difficulty concentrating, and challenges with problem-solving. Patients may notice that they struggle to recall recent events or find it increasingly difficult to follow conversations. Additionally, changes in mood or behavior, such as increased irritability or withdrawal from social activities, can signal the onset of dementia. These early signs can often be mistaken for normal aging or stress, making awareness crucial for timely intervention.

Diagnosing early onset dementia typically involves a comprehensive assessment by healthcare professionals. This process often starts with a detailed medical history and a physical examination to rule out other medical conditions that could mimic dementia symptoms. Cognitive tests are commonly administered to evaluate memory, attention, and problem-solving abilities. Healthcare providers may also use brain imaging techniques, such as MRI or CT scans, to identify any structural changes in the brain that may indicate dementia.

It's important for patients and their caregivers to recognize that early diagnosis can significantly impact the course of the disease. Early intervention allows for better planning and management of symptoms, including access to therapies that may slow progression. It also helps patients and families prepare for the future, enabling them to make informed decisions regarding care and support. Engaging with healthcare providers about symptoms as soon as they arise can facilitate timely diagnosis and intervention.

In addition to medical evaluations, keeping a symptom diary can be beneficial for both patients and healthcare providers. This diary can record changes in cognition, mood, and daily functioning, providing a clearer picture of the individual's experience over time. Such documentation can also help caregivers articulate their observations during medical appointments, ensuring that all relevant information is communicated effectively. This collaborative approach between patients, caregivers, and medical professionals is essential for accurate diagnosis and tailored care plans.

As research continues to evolve in the field of dementia, understanding symptoms and obtaining an accurate diagnosis remains a pivotal step for those affected. Patients are encouraged to stay informed about the latest developments, including clinical trials and emerging therapies. Engaging with support groups and resources can also provide valuable insights and enhance the overall quality of life. By recognizing symptoms early and seeking a proper diagnosis, individuals can take proactive steps towards managing their condition and maintaining their well-being.

The Impact of Early Onset Dementia

The impact of early onset dementia can be profound, affecting not only the individuals diagnosed but also their families, caregivers, and communities. Early onset dementia, defined as dementia occurring before the age of 65, can present unique challenges that differ from those experienced by older individuals. Patients may experience a range of symptoms including memory loss, cognitive decline, and changes in mood or behavior, often while still navigating personal and professional responsibilities. This can lead to significant emotional distress, not only for the patients but also for loved ones who may struggle to understand and cope with the changes.

Caregiving for those with early onset dementia can be particularly demanding. Family members often take on the role of caregivers, which may require them to balance their own work, personal lives, and caregiving responsibilities. The emotional and physical toll can be substantial, leading to caregiver burnout. It is crucial for caregivers to seek support, whether through local support groups, online communities, or professional counseling. Understanding the symptoms and progression of early onset dementia can help caregivers manage their expectations and develop effective strategies for providing care while maintaining their own well-being.

Engagement in meaningful activities is essential for individuals living with early onset dementia, as it can enhance their quality of life and slow cognitive decline. Dementia-friendly activities, such as art therapy, music, or gentle exercise, can foster social interaction and stimulate cognitive functions. Encouraging involvement in hobbies and interests can also provide a sense of purpose and identity, helping patients to retain aspects of their former selves. It's important for caregivers to create an environment that promotes engagement, ensuring that activities are tailored to the individual's abilities and preferences.

Nutrition plays a crucial role in the management of dementia. A balanced diet rich in fruits, vegetables, whole grains, and healthy fats can support brain health and overall well-being. Certain nutrients, such as omega-3 fatty acids and antioxidants, have been linked to cognitive function and may help delay the progression of symptoms. Caregivers should be mindful of the dietary needs of those with early onset dementia, considering meal planning and preparation as an opportunity for engagement. Involving patients in cooking can not only enhance their nutritional intake but also provide a comforting routine.

As early onset dementia progresses, legal and financial planning becomes increasingly important. Individuals and families must address issues such as power of attorney, healthcare directives, and financial management. Proactive planning can alleviate stress and ensure that patients' wishes are honored as their condition evolves. Additionally, staying informed about ongoing dementia research and clinical trials can provide hope and potential avenues for treatment. Engaging with healthcare professionals, legal advisors, and support organizations can empower patients and families to navigate this complex journey with confidence and clarity.

Chapter 2: Living Well with Dementia

Embracing the Diagnosis

Embracing a diagnosis of early onset dementia can be a challenging and emotional journey. It is natural to experience a myriad of feelings upon receiving this diagnosis, including fear, confusion, and sadness. However, accepting the reality of the situation is a crucial step toward managing your health and well-being. Understanding what early onset dementia means and how it can affect your life is essential in beginning to navigate this new path. This knowledge allows you to seek appropriate support and resources tailored to your needs.

As you acclimate to your diagnosis, it is important to recognize the value of a strong support network. Engaging with family, friends, and support groups can provide emotional relief and practical assistance. These connections can help alleviate feelings of isolation that often accompany a dementia diagnosis. Caregivers play a vital role in this process, as they can offer understanding, companionship, and the necessary help for daily activities. Open communication with loved ones about your feelings and needs can foster a supportive environment that promotes emotional well-being.

Incorporating dementia-friendly activities into your daily routine can significantly improve your quality of life. These activities, which might include arts and crafts, gardening, or simple games, not only provide enjoyment but also stimulate cognitive function and enhance social interaction. Finding hobbies that resonate with your interests can create a sense of purpose and fulfillment. Additionally, engaging in physical activities tailored to your abilities can further boost your mood and overall health, contributing to a more positive living experience.

Nutrition plays a pivotal role in managing early onset dementia and can impact cognitive health. Adopting a well-balanced diet rich in fruits, vegetables, whole grains, and healthy fats is essential. Foods high in antioxidants and omega-3 fatty acids, such as fish and nuts, may provide protective benefits for brain health. Staying hydrated and maintaining a regular eating schedule can also support cognitive function. Collaborating with a nutritionist familiar with dementia care can help you create a personalized meal plan that addresses your nutritional needs while also considering any preferences or dietary restrictions you may have.

Finally, embracing your diagnosis means being proactive about legal and financial planning. Understanding your rights and options regarding healthcare decisions, power of attorney, and advanced directives is crucial. It is advisable to consult with professionals who specialize in elder law and financial planning for individuals with dementia. Additionally, staying informed about ongoing dementia research and clinical trials can open doors to new treatments and therapies. This proactive approach not only empowers you but also ensures that your wishes and needs are respected as you navigate this journey.

Strategies for Daily Living

Living with early onset dementia necessitates adjustments to daily routines that can enhance quality of life and promote independence. One effective strategy is establishing a consistent daily schedule. A structured routine helps minimize confusion and anxiety, as patients can anticipate what comes next. This consistency can include regular times for meals, exercise, and social activities. Caregivers can assist by creating visual schedules or checklists, which serve as reminders for daily tasks, thus fostering a sense of accomplishment and control.

Engagement in meaningful activities is crucial for cognitive stimulation and emotional well-being. Patients should be encouraged to pursue hobbies and interests that bring joy and fulfillment. Simple activities such as gardening, painting, or engaging in puzzles can stimulate the mind and provide a sense of purpose. Social interactions are equally important; participating in group activities or support groups can help mitigate feelings of isolation. Caregivers can facilitate these engagements by organizing small gatherings or coordinating participation in community events, thus ensuring that patients remain socially connected.

Nutrition plays a vital role in managing health, and a well-balanced diet can positively impact cognitive function. Incorporating foods rich in omega-3 fatty acids, antioxidants, and vitamins can support brain health. Caregivers should focus on preparing meals that are not only nutritious but also appealing to the patient's tastes. Meal planning can be a collaborative effort, allowing patients to participate in choosing meals, which fosters independence and enjoyment. Additionally, keeping hydrated is essential; caregivers should encourage regular fluid intake throughout the day.

Technology can serve as a valuable tool in daily living for individuals with early onset dementia. Utilizing smart home devices can enhance safety and convenience, allowing patients to maintain independence. For instance, voice-activated assistants can help with reminders for medications or appointments. There are also apps designed to aid memory, organization, and communication. Caregivers can help patients learn to use these technologies, ensuring they are equipped to navigate their daily lives more effectively and confidently.

Finally, communication strategies are crucial in fostering understanding and connection between patients and their caregivers. It is important for caregivers to use clear, simple language and to maintain a calm and patient demeanor. Active listening and validating feelings can enhance the relationship and reduce frustration. Non-verbal cues, such as gestures and facial expressions, can also play a significant role in communication. By creating an environment where patients feel heard and understood, caregivers can significantly improve the overall quality of daily interactions, promoting a sense of trust and emotional security.

Building a Support Network

Building a support network is essential for individuals living with early onset dementia. A support network can significantly enhance the quality of life and emotional well-being of patients and their caregivers. Such a network typically includes family, friends, healthcare providers, dementia support groups, and community resources. Connecting with others who understand the challenges of dementia can provide emotional comfort, practical assistance, and valuable information. Establishing and nurturing these relationships can empower patients to cope better with their condition and maintain a sense of normalcy in their lives.

Family members often serve as the first line of support for individuals with early onset dementia. Communicating openly with family about the diagnosis can create a foundation of understanding and compassion. It is important for families to educate themselves on dementia to better grasp the changes their loved one is experiencing. Organizing family meetings to discuss care strategies, emotional needs, and daily challenges can foster a collaborative approach to caregiving. This not only strengthens familial bonds but also ensures that everyone is on the same page regarding the patient's care and support.

In addition to family, joining a support group can be immensely beneficial. Support groups provide a safe space for individuals with dementia to share their experiences, feelings, and coping strategies. Many of these groups are facilitated by professionals or trained volunteers who can guide discussions and offer insights. Participants often find solace in knowing they are not alone in their journey. Additionally, these groups can introduce patients and caregivers to various resources, such as educational materials, workshops, and local services that cater specifically to the needs of people affected by dementia.

Community resources also play a crucial role in building a robust support network. Local organizations, such as Alzheimer's associations or health departments, often provide programs tailored to individuals with dementia and their caregivers. These resources may include recreational activities, educational seminars, and respite care options. Engaging in dementia-friendly activities can enhance social interaction and cognitive stimulation, which are vital for maintaining mental and emotional health. By participating in these community programs, patients can connect with others and create friendships that can last a lifetime.

Lastly, leveraging technology can further enhance a support network. Numerous apps and online platforms are designed to assist dementia patients and their caregivers in managing daily tasks, tracking symptoms, and organizing appointments. Virtual support groups and forums can connect individuals with others across the globe, expanding their network beyond local resources. Additionally, technology can facilitate communication with family and friends, allowing patients to maintain relationships even when in-person visits are challenging. By combining these various elements—family, support groups, community resources, and technology—individuals with early onset dementia can create a comprehensive support network that nurtures their emotional and practical needs.

Chapter 3: Caregiver Support

Understanding the Role of Caregivers

Understanding the role of caregivers is essential for individuals living with early onset dementia. Caregivers are often family members or close friends who provide the necessary support and assistance to maintain the quality of life for those affected by dementia. They play a critical role in managing daily activities, ensuring safety, and facilitating communication. Understanding this dynamic can help patients and caregivers alike navigate the challenges of dementia more effectively.

Caregivers fulfill a variety of responsibilities that extend beyond physical assistance. They often coordinate medical appointments, manage medications, and advocate for the patient's needs within healthcare settings. This role requires a deep understanding of the patient's condition, as well as the ability to adapt to changing needs. By recognizing the multifaceted nature of caregiving, patients can engage more meaningfully with their caregivers, fostering a collaborative environment that enhances both care and emotional support.

Emotional support is another vital aspect of caregiving. Caregivers often experience stress, anxiety, and feelings of isolation as they navigate their responsibilities. Patients can help alleviate some of this burden by maintaining open lines of communication. Expressing needs, preferences, and feelings can strengthen the caregiver-patient relationship and promote mutual understanding. Additionally, caregivers benefit from emotional support networks, which can provide them with resources and encouragement, reinforcing the importance of self-care.

Engaging in dementia-friendly activities is an important way for patients and caregivers to connect. Shared activities can promote cognitive engagement and emotional well-being, helping to mitigate some symptoms of dementia. These activities can range from simple puzzles and games to more involved projects like gardening or art. Caregivers can play a pivotal role in identifying and facilitating these activities, ensuring they are enjoyable and tailored to the patient's abilities and interests.

Lastly, caregivers can assist with practical matters such as nutrition and legal planning. A balanced diet is crucial for maintaining health, and caregivers can help prepare meals that align with dietary recommendations for dementia prevention. They can also support discussions about legal and financial planning, ensuring that patients' wishes are respected as their condition progresses. By understanding the comprehensive role caregivers play, patients can better appreciate their contributions and work together to create a supportive and enriching environment.

Resources for Caregiver Support

As individuals living with early onset dementia, having a reliable support system is crucial for managing daily challenges and maintaining quality of life. Caregivers play an integral role in this journey, often providing emotional, physical, and logistical support. To empower both patients and their caregivers, various resources can be accessed to enhance caregiving experiences and knowledge. These resources not only promote a better understanding of dementia but also offer practical tools to improve care and support.

Numerous organizations and associations focus on dementia care support, providing educational materials, workshops, and training for caregivers. The Alzheimer's Association and the Dementia Society of America, for example, offer comprehensive resources that include online webinars, local support groups, and informational brochures. These organizations facilitate connections with other caregivers, allowing them to share experiences, tips, and emotional support, which can be invaluable when navigating the complexities of dementia care.

Technology has become a significant ally in caregiving, with various apps and devices designed to assist both caregivers and patients. These tools can help manage daily schedules, medication reminders, and communication aids, simplifying the caregiving process. For instance, wearable devices can monitor health metrics and alert caregivers in case of emergencies, thereby enhancing safety. By incorporating technology into caregiving, caregivers can focus more on meaningful interactions with patients rather than on logistics.

Nutrition plays a pivotal role in supporting brain health and overall well-being. Caregivers should be equipped with knowledge about diets that may benefit individuals with dementia, such as the Mediterranean diet, which emphasizes fruits, vegetables, whole grains, and healthy fats. Resources such as nutrition workshops, cookbooks, and meal-planning guides can support caregivers in preparing meals that are not only nutritious but also appealing to those with dietary restrictions or specific preferences. Engaging patients in meal preparation can also serve as a bonding activity, enriching their daily experience.

Lastly, understanding the legal and financial aspects of dementia care is essential for both patients and their caregivers. Resources that provide information on power of attorney, advance directives, and financial planning can help ease the stress of making important decisions. Legal aid organizations often offer consultations and materials to guide families through these processes, ensuring that both caregivers and patients feel secure and informed. By utilizing these resources, caregivers can focus on providing compassionate care while navigating the complexities associated with dementia.

Communication Between Patients and Caregivers

Effective communication between patients and caregivers is vital for ensuring that the needs of individuals living with early onset dementia are met. This relationship is built on trust and understanding, allowing for smoother interactions and fostering a supportive environment. Patients often experience challenges in expressing their thoughts and feelings, which can lead to frustration. Caregivers must develop keen listening skills and patience to decipher non-verbal cues and to provide reassurance. By creating an atmosphere where patients feel safe to share their concerns, caregivers can significantly enhance the quality of care.

One crucial aspect of communication is the use of clear and simple language. Caregivers should avoid complex phrases and jargon that may confuse patients. Instead, using short sentences and familiar terms can help convey messages more effectively. Visual aids, such as pictures or written notes, can also support understanding. This approach not only facilitates better communication but also empowers patients to engage in conversations about their care preferences, thereby encouraging their autonomy and involvement in decision-making.

Non-verbal communication plays a significant role in interactions with dementia patients. Body language, facial expressions, and tone of voice can all convey emotions and intentions. Caregivers should be mindful of their own non-verbal cues, as well as those of the patient. A warm smile or gentle touch can provide comfort and reassurance, while a tense posture may lead to anxiety. Recognizing and responding to these non-verbal signals can strengthen the bond between patients and caregivers, making it easier to navigate challenging moments.

In addition to verbal and non-verbal communication, establishing routines can enhance the interaction between patients and caregivers. Predictable schedules can help patients feel more secure and reduce confusion, allowing for easier communication. Caregivers can incorporate regular check-ins and discussions about daily activities, providing opportunities for patients to express their thoughts and feelings. This consistent approach not only fosters a sense of stability but also opens up channels for communication, making it easier for caregivers to address any concerns that may arise.

Lastly, incorporating technology can significantly improve communication between patients and caregivers. Tools such as communication apps, reminder systems, and video calls can bridge gaps created by cognitive decline. These technologies can help patients remember important information, stay connected with loved ones, and engage in activities that stimulate cognitive function. Caregivers should explore and utilize these tools to enhance their communication strategies, ultimately leading to a more enriching experience for both parties involved in the caregiving journey.

Chapter 4: Engaging in Dementia-Friendly Activities

Importance of Engagement

Engagement is a crucial aspect of maintaining quality of life for individuals living with early onset dementia. It involves participating in various activities that stimulate the mind, encourage social interaction, and foster a sense of purpose. Engaging in meaningful activities can help alleviate feelings of isolation and depression, which are common among dementia patients. By prioritizing engagement, patients can benefit from improved cognitive function, enhanced emotional well-being, and a greater sense of connection with their loved ones and the community.

Social engagement is particularly important for individuals with early onset dementia. Participating in group activities, whether through support groups, community events, or recreational classes, can create opportunities for building relationships and sharing experiences. These interactions can provide emotional support and reduce the stigma that often accompanies dementia. Engaging with others who understand the challenges of living with dementia can foster camaraderie and help patients feel less alone in their journey.

Cognitive engagement, such as puzzles, games, and art activities, plays a significant role in stimulating the brain. These activities can help maintain cognitive function and delay the progression of symptoms. Simple tasks like reading, writing, or even gardening can serve as beneficial forms of mental exercise. Caregivers can assist by introducing dementia-friendly activities that are tailored to the individual's interests and capabilities, ensuring that engagement remains enjoyable and fulfilling rather than overwhelming.

Physical engagement is another critical component of overall well-being. Regular physical activity, tailored to the individual's abilities, can enhance physical health and improve mood. Activities such as walking, dancing, or gentle yoga not only promote physical fitness but also encourage social interaction when done in groups. Caregivers should consider incorporating movement-based activities into daily routines, as the benefits of physical engagement extend beyond fitness to include enhanced cognitive and emotional health.

Lastly, engagement extends to the use of technology, which can serve as a valuable tool for enhancing communication and connection. Numerous apps and devices are designed to support individuals with dementia, offering reminders, facilitating social interactions, and even providing entertainment. Embracing technology can empower patients to maintain independence and engage with their environment more effectively. By recognizing the importance of engagement in all its forms, patients and caregivers can work together to create a supportive and enriching environment, leading to a more fulfilling life despite the challenges of early onset dementia.

Activities for Cognitive Stimulation

Engaging in cognitive stimulation activities is crucial for individuals with early onset dementia, as these activities can help maintain mental acuity and enhance overall well-being. Cognitive stimulation refers to a range of activities designed to encourage thinking, memory, and problem-solving skills. Simple exercises such as puzzles, word games, or even memory matching games can provide an enjoyable way to challenge the brain. These activities not only foster cognitive engagement but also promote social interaction, which can be particularly beneficial for emotional health.

Incorporating daily routines that include cognitive stimulation can make a significant difference in the lives of dementia patients. For instance, setting aside specific times for reading, engaging in arts and crafts, or playing board games can establish a comforting routine. Caregivers can play an essential role in this process by participating in these activities and encouraging their loved ones to join in. Such involvement can foster a sense of normalcy and continuity, which is often comforting for those facing the challenges of early onset dementia.

Technology can also serve as a valuable tool for cognitive stimulation. Various applications and online platforms offer games and exercises tailored for individuals experiencing cognitive decline. These tools often come with engaging graphics and interactive elements that can capture the attention of users. Moreover, technology can facilitate virtual connections with family and friends, allowing for social engagement and cognitive challenges through shared activities, such as online trivia games or virtual book clubs.

Another effective approach is to incorporate reminiscence therapy into cognitive stimulation activities. This involves engaging in discussions about past experiences, memories, and significant life events. Caregivers can use photo albums, music, or familiar objects to spark memories and facilitate conversations. This not only helps in stimulating cognitive functions but also strengthens emotional bonds between the patient and caregiver, creating a supportive environment essential for mental health.

Lastly, it's important to recognize the role of nutrition in cognitive health. A balanced diet rich in antioxidants, omega-3 fatty acids, and vitamins can support brain function. Caregivers should consider incorporating foods like fruits, vegetables, fish, and nuts into meals while also involving patients in meal planning or cooking as a way to stimulate cognitive skills. This approach not only promotes better nutrition but also engages patients in meaningful activities, leading to a holistic strategy for managing early onset dementia.

Social Activities and Community Involvement

Social activities and community involvement play a vital role in enhancing the quality of life for individuals living with early onset dementia. Engaging in social activities helps combat feelings of isolation and loneliness that can often accompany the condition. These activities provide opportunities for meaningful interactions, which are essential for emotional well-being. Joining clubs, participating in group outings, or attending community events can foster a sense of belonging and purpose, making daily life more enjoyable and fulfilling.

Participating in community activities can also help dementia patients maintain cognitive function. Engaging in puzzles, arts and crafts, or games that require problem-solving can stimulate the brain and encourage social interaction. Many communities offer programs specifically designed for individuals with cognitive impairments, creating a safe and supportive environment for participation. These programs not only promote mental engagement but also allow patients to connect with others who may share similar experiences, thereby reducing stigma and enhancing social networks.

Involvement in social activities can also benefit caregivers. By encouraging patients to engage with their peers, caregivers can take much-needed breaks, reducing their stress and preventing burnout. Community programs often provide resources and support for caregivers, allowing them to learn new strategies for managing their loved ones' care. This dual benefit highlights the importance of fostering community connections not just for patients, but also for their caregivers, promoting an overall supportive ecosystem.

Additionally, local organizations and support groups can be invaluable resources for patients and caregivers alike. These groups often host workshops, seminars, and events focused on dementia education, enabling participants to gain knowledge about the condition and learn effective coping strategies. Through these gatherings, individuals can share their experiences, exchange information about available resources, and build lasting relationships that provide emotional support.

Finally, technology can play a significant role in enhancing social activities and community involvement. Many platforms now offer virtual meet-ups, allowing individuals with early onset dementia to connect with others from the comfort of their homes. These online communities can serve as a lifeline for those who may have mobility issues or prefer staying indoors. By utilizing technology, patients can maintain their social connections and continue to engage with the world around them, ensuring that they remain active participants in their communities.

Chapter 5: Nutrition and Diet for Dementia Prevention

Foods That Support Brain Health

Foods that support brain health play a crucial role in managing early onset dementia and enhancing the quality of life for those affected by it. A balanced and nutritious diet can help improve cognitive function and potentially slow the progression of dementia symptoms. Incorporating specific foods into daily meals can provide essential nutrients that support brain health, making it easier for patients to engage in activities and maintain independence.

One of the most beneficial food groups for brain health is fatty fish, such as salmon, mackerel, and sardines. These fish are rich in omega-3 fatty acids, which are vital for maintaining the structure and function of brain cells. Omega-3s have been shown to improve memory and cognitive performance, making them an essential addition to the diet of individuals experiencing cognitive decline. Regular consumption of fatty fish can also reduce inflammation and promote overall cardiovascular health, which is closely linked to brain function.

Fruits and vegetables, particularly those that are deeply colored, are also important for supporting brain health. Berries, such as blueberries and strawberries, are high in antioxidants that help protect brain cells from oxidative stress. Leafy greens like spinach and kale are packed with vitamins and minerals that contribute to cognitive function. Including a variety of these colorful fruits and vegetables in meals can provide essential nutrients that support mental clarity and emotional well-being.

Whole grains are another key component of a brain-healthy diet. Foods such as quinoa, brown rice, and whole-grain bread are rich in fiber and help regulate blood sugar levels. Stable blood sugar is essential for maintaining energy and focus throughout the day.

Additionally, whole grains provide B vitamins, which play a critical role in brain health by supporting the production of neurotransmitters that facilitate communication between brain cells.

Lastly, nuts and seeds, particularly walnuts and flaxseeds, are excellent sources of nutrients that promote cognitive health. These foods are rich in vitamin E, an antioxidant that has been linked to a lower risk of cognitive decline. Incorporating a handful of nuts or seeds into snacks or meals can provide a convenient way to boost brain health. By focusing on a diet rich in these brain-boosting foods, individuals with early onset dementia can support their cognitive function and improve their overall quality of life.

Meal Planning and Preparation

Meal planning and preparation are essential components of maintaining a healthy lifestyle, especially for individuals living with early onset dementia. A well-structured meal plan not only ensures nutritional needs are met but also aids in maintaining cognitive function and emotional well-being. Creating a weekly menu can help reduce the stress of last-minute decisions about food, which can be overwhelming for both patients and caregivers. It is beneficial to involve the individual in the planning process to foster a sense of independence and ownership over their meals.

When planning meals, it is important to focus on a balanced diet rich in fruits, vegetables, whole grains, lean proteins, and healthy fats. Foods high in antioxidants, omega-3 fatty acids, and vitamins can support brain health and may slow the progression of cognitive decline. Caregivers should consider dietary preferences, allergies, and any specific health conditions when designing meal plans. Incorporating familiar recipes can also trigger pleasant memories and promote engagement during mealtime, creating a positive atmosphere around food.

Preparation techniques can significantly impact the ease of mealtime routines. Batch cooking and freezing meals in advance can alleviate the daily pressure of cooking, making it simpler to provide nutritious options. Using simple recipes with minimal ingredients can help maintain focus and reduce confusion. Caregivers can also set up a designated cooking space equipped with easy-to-use tools and appliances to make the process more manageable. Engaging the individual in the preparation can provide a sense of purpose and stimulate cognitive function through hands-on activity.

Incorporating technology can further enhance meal planning and preparation. There are various apps designed to assist with grocery lists, meal ideas, and even dietary tracking. Smart kitchen devices can simplify cooking processes; for instance, slow cookers and programmable ovens can be set to prepare meals with minimal supervision. Voice-activated assistants can provide reminders for meal times or guide users through simple recipes, fostering independence and confidence in the kitchen.

Lastly, it is crucial to create a supportive dining environment that promotes social interaction and enjoyment during meals. Eating together, whether with family, friends, or caregivers, can enhance the experience and encourage better eating habits. Establishing regular meal times and maintaining consistency in routines can also provide structure, which is beneficial for individuals with dementia. By prioritizing meal planning and preparation, caregivers can significantly contribute to the quality of life for those living with early onset dementia, ensuring that nutritious meals are both accessible and enjoyable.

The Role of Hydration

The role of hydration in the well-being of individuals with early onset dementia cannot be overstated. Proper hydration is essential for maintaining overall health and cognitive function. Water plays a crucial role in numerous bodily processes, including digestion, circulation, and temperature regulation. For dementia patients, staying hydrated can help alleviate some common symptoms, such as confusion and fatigue, which can exacerbate the challenges they already face. It is important for caregivers and patients alike to understand the significance of regular fluid intake and its impact on both physical and mental health.

Dehydration can lead to serious complications, especially in individuals with early onset dementia. Symptoms of dehydration may mimic or worsen cognitive impairment, leading to increased confusion or agitation. This can create a cycle of misunderstanding, where caregivers may mistakenly attribute behavioral changes to the progression of dementia rather than a simple lack of hydration. Recognizing early signs of dehydration, such as dry mouth, decreased urine output, or headaches, is vital for timely intervention and care.

Incorporating hydration into daily routines is essential for both patients and caregivers. Caregivers should encourage frequent water breaks and provide a variety of fluids, including water, herbal teas, and broths, to keep hydration interesting and appealing. Additionally, incorporating hydrating foods, such as fruits and vegetables, into meals can contribute to overall fluid intake. Making hydration a part of meal planning not only ensures adequate fluid intake but also promotes a more balanced and nutritious diet, which is crucial for overall health in dementia management.

Creating dementia-friendly environments can further support hydration efforts. Placing water bottles or glasses in easily accessible locations serves as a visual reminder for patients to drink more fluids throughout the day. Caregivers can also establish regular hydration times, such as during meals or while watching television, to help patients develop a routine. Using technology, such as reminders on smartphones or tablets, can assist in promoting hydration habits, making it easier for both caregivers and patients to stay on track.

Finally, fostering open communication about hydration needs is important for effective care. Caregivers should feel comfortable discussing hydration with healthcare providers, especially if there are concerns about the patient's fluid intake or related health issues.

Understanding the individual hydration needs of dementia patients can lead to better health outcomes and improve quality of life. By prioritizing hydration and making it an integral part of daily care plans, caregivers can significantly enhance the well-being of individuals living with early onset dementia.

Chapter 6: Utilizing Technology Aids

Overview of Technology for Dementia Care

Technology has become an essential component in the care and support of individuals living with dementia, particularly for those experiencing early onset dementia. Innovations in this field aim to enhance the quality of life for patients and provide caregivers with valuable tools to assist them in daily activities. From communication devices to monitoring systems, the array of technology available today is designed to foster independence while ensuring safety and support for individuals navigating the challenges of dementia.

One significant area of technological advancement is the development of communication aids. These tools help bridge the gap between patients and their loved ones, facilitating meaningful interactions. Applications on smartphones and tablets can simplify communication by using visual cues, reminders, and easy-to-navigate interfaces. Additionally, specialized devices exist that convert speech to text and vice versa, allowing for clearer dialogue and reducing frustration for both patients and caregivers. Such technologies not only improve communication but also support emotional connections, which are vital for mental health.

Monitoring technologies, including wearable devices and home sensors, have emerged as critical tools for ensuring the safety of individuals with dementia. Wearables can track vital signs and detect falls, alerting caregivers or emergency services if necessary. Home sensors can monitor movement patterns, enabling caregivers to receive notifications if unusual behavior is detected, such as wandering or inactivity. These technologies provide peace of mind for families, knowing that their loved ones are being monitored effectively, which allows for a greater sense of autonomy for patients.

Engagement technologies play a pivotal role in promoting cognitive health and providing meaningful activities for individuals with dementia. Applications designed with dementia-friendly interfaces offer puzzles, games, and memory exercises tailored to various cognitive levels. Virtual reality experiences can transport users to familiar places or stimulate conversation through shared experiences. Such engagement not only helps maintain cognitive function but also encourages social interaction, reducing feelings of isolation that many dementia patients may encounter.

As technology continues to evolve, it is essential for patients, families, and caregivers to stay informed about the latest advancements that could enhance care and support. Understanding the range of available options empowers individuals to make informed decisions about their care strategies. By embracing technology, those affected by early onset dementia can benefit from enhanced communication, increased safety, and improved engagement, ultimately leading to a better quality of life.

Apps for Daily Living

Apps designed for daily living can play a significant role in enhancing the quality of life for individuals with early onset dementia. These applications offer a variety of tools that can assist with memory support, organization, and daily tasks, making it easier for patients to navigate their day-to-day activities. By leveraging technology, individuals can maintain a sense of independence while also staying connected with caregivers and loved ones. The right apps can help with scheduling, reminders, and even cognitive exercises, ultimately fostering a greater sense of control and stability.

One of the most beneficial types of apps for daily living are those focused on reminders and scheduling. Calendar applications can help users keep track of important appointments and daily tasks, while reminder apps can send notifications for medications, meals, and other essential activities. This can alleviate anxiety for both patients and caregivers, as it reduces the burden of remembering every detail.

Many of these apps are customizable, allowing users to set alarms and notifications that suit their unique routines and preferences.

In addition to scheduling and reminders, cognitive training apps can provide engaging activities that stimulate mental functions. These apps often include puzzles, memory games, and brain teasers designed to challenge cognitive abilities, which can be particularly beneficial for maintaining mental agility in the face of early onset dementia. Regular use of these cognitive exercises can help slow cognitive decline and promote a sense of achievement and satisfaction. Caregivers can also encourage participation in these activities, turning them into fun and interactive sessions that strengthen their bond.

Another area where apps can assist is in communication. Social connection is vital for emotional well-being, and there are various apps that facilitate easier communication with family and friends. Video calling and messaging platforms allow patients to maintain relationships despite any physical limitations. Additionally, there are apps designed specifically for individuals with speech difficulties, offering alternative communication methods that can enhance interaction and engagement. These tools can significantly reduce feelings of isolation and promote a supportive network, which is essential for emotional health.

Lastly, many apps focus on nutrition and wellness, providing recipes, meal planning, and dietary tracking to support a healthy lifestyle. Proper nutrition is known to play a role in brain health, and apps can help users make informed choices about their diets. By offering easy-to-follow recipes and allowing users to track their daily intake, these applications can empower individuals with early onset dementia to take charge of their nutritional needs. Caregivers can also utilize these tools to ensure that meals are balanced and cater to any specific dietary requirements, promoting overall well-being.

Safety and Monitoring Devices

Safety and monitoring devices play an essential role in enhancing the quality of life for individuals living with early onset dementia. These devices are designed to assist both patients and caregivers by providing real-time information and support, helping to alleviate some of the anxiety and challenges associated with memory loss. As dementia progresses, the risk of accidents or wandering can increase, making it crucial to have tools in place that promote safety and independence. From alert systems to smart home technologies, understanding the options available can empower patients and caregivers alike.

One of the most common safety devices is a personal emergency response system (PERS). This technology allows individuals to call for help at the push of a button, offering peace of mind for both patients and their loved ones. In many cases, these devices can be worn as pendants or wristbands, making them easy to access in emergencies. Moreover, some advanced systems are equipped with fall detection features that automatically notify caregivers or emergency services if a fall is detected, further enhancing safety measures for those living with dementia.

Smart home technology has also emerged as a valuable resource for individuals with early onset dementia. Devices such as smart door locks, motion sensors, and surveillance cameras can help monitor the home environment while allowing patients to maintain a sense of independence. For instance, motion sensors can alert caregivers if a patient leaves a designated area, providing timely information that can prevent wandering. Additionally, smart home assistants can help with daily tasks, reminding patients of appointments, medications, or even social activities, fostering engagement and reducing feelings of isolation.

Incorporating technology aids into daily routines can also support cognitive function and mental health. For example, digital calendars or reminder apps can help patients keep track of important dates and encourage regular engagement in activities they enjoy, which is vital for emotional well-being. Furthermore, there are numerous applications designed specifically for dementia care, offering brain games and memory exercises that can stimulate cognitive abilities while making the process enjoyable. These tools not only enhance safety but also contribute to a more fulfilling daily experience.

It is important to consider that while safety and monitoring devices can significantly improve the living conditions for those with early onset dementia, they should be used in conjunction with a comprehensive care plan tailored to individual needs. Open communication between patients, caregivers, and healthcare providers is essential to determine which devices will be most beneficial. By integrating these technologies thoughtfully, caregivers can create a supportive environment that promotes autonomy while ensuring safety, ultimately leading to a better quality of life for individuals affected by dementia.

Chapter 7: Legal and Financial Planning

Importance of Early Planning

Early planning plays a crucial role in managing early onset dementia, providing patients and their families with a roadmap for navigating the challenges that lie ahead. As the diagnosis becomes a reality, it is essential to recognize that early intervention not only improves the quality of life but also empowers individuals to maintain a sense of control over their future. By addressing various aspects such as legal, financial, and healthcare considerations, patients can create a comprehensive plan that serves their needs and preferences throughout their journey with dementia.

One significant advantage of early planning is the ability to make informed decisions while cognitive abilities are still relatively intact. Engaging in discussions about healthcare preferences, treatment options, and end-of-life care can alleviate the stress and confusion that often accompany these topics later in the disease progression. Setting up advanced directives and durable powers of attorney ensures that patients' wishes are respected, providing peace of mind for both the individual and their loved ones. This proactive approach allows for open communication, which is essential in fostering an environment of support and understanding.

In addition to legal and healthcare planning, early preparation can also extend to financial matters. Understanding the potential costs associated with dementia care is vital, as it enables families to budget appropriately and explore available resources. This includes researching insurance options, government assistance programs, and community resources that may offer financial support. By establishing a clear financial plan, patients can alleviate some of the burdens on their caregivers, allowing them to focus on providing emotional support and facilitating meaningful engagement in daily activities.

Furthermore, early planning encourages the incorporation of lifestyle changes that can promote overall well-being. Nutrition and diet play a significant role in brain health, and by prioritizing a balanced diet rich in antioxidants, healthy fats, and essential nutrients, patients can potentially slow cognitive decline. Additionally, engaging in dementia-friendly activities tailored to individual interests not only fosters a sense of purpose but also enhances social interactions and mental stimulation. These proactive steps contribute to a healthier, more fulfilling life while living with early onset dementia.

Finally, leveraging technology aids can significantly enhance the quality of life for individuals with dementia. From medication reminders to communication tools, technology can assist in maintaining independence and safety. Early planning allows patients and caregivers to explore various technological solutions that cater to specific needs, ensuring that they are equipped with the right tools as the condition progresses. By addressing these aspects early on, individuals can lead a more empowered and fulfilling life, emphasizing the importance of taking proactive steps in the face of early onset dementia.

Legal Documents to Consider

Legal documents play a crucial role in ensuring that individuals with early onset dementia have their preferences and wishes respected as their condition progresses. It is vital for dementia patients to consider establishing a power of attorney, which grants a trusted person the authority to make financial and legal decisions on their behalf. This document is particularly important as it allows patients to designate someone who understands their values and goals, ensuring that their best interests are upheld even when they may no longer be able to express them.

Another essential legal document is a living will. This document outlines specific medical treatments an individual does or does not wish to receive in the event they become unable to communicate their preferences. It is essential for dementia patients to discuss their wishes regarding end-of-life care with family members and healthcare providers. Having a living will in place can alleviate confusion and stress for caregivers and loved ones, allowing them to make informed decisions that align with the patient's values.

Advance healthcare directives are also significant for those living with early onset dementia. These directives allow individuals to specify their medical treatment preferences and appoint a healthcare proxy who will make decisions on their behalf if they become incapacitated. By discussing these topics early, patients can ensure that their healthcare choices are respected even as their cognitive abilities decline. Furthermore, these directives can help to ease the burden on caregivers, who may struggle with making difficult decisions in emotionally charged situations.

In addition to these documents, patients should consider updating their wills and trusts. As life circumstances change, including the progression of dementia, it is essential to revisit and possibly revise estate planning documents. This ensures that assets are distributed according to the patient's wishes and provides clarity for family members. Consulting with an attorney who specializes in elder law or estate planning can help ensure that all necessary considerations are addressed, and that the legal documents reflect the patient's current needs and desires.

Finally, it is advisable for dementia patients to keep all legal documents organized and accessible. Maintaining a central file that includes copies of the power of attorney, living will, advance healthcare directive, and any other relevant legal documents can simplify the process for caregivers and family members. Regularly reviewing and updating these documents as needed is important to reflect any changes in preferences or circumstances. By taking these proactive steps, individuals with early onset dementia can secure their rights and preferences, ensuring peace of mind for themselves and their loved ones.

Managing Finances and Resources

Managing finances and resources is a crucial aspect of living well with early onset dementia. As the condition progresses, individuals may find it increasingly challenging to handle financial responsibilities, making it essential to establish a clear strategy. This involves organizing important documents, understanding income sources, and identifying necessary expenses. Creating a budget can help ensure that financial resources are allocated effectively, allowing for essential needs such as housing, healthcare, and daily living expenses to be met while preserving quality of life.

Involving trusted family members or caregivers in financial management can alleviate some of the stress associated with handling finances alone. Open communication about financial matters is vital, as it allows caregivers to support the individual effectively. Setting up joint accounts or designated financial power of attorney can provide additional security and oversight. This collaborative approach not only enhances accountability but also ensures that financial decisions reflect the individual's values and preferences.

Exploring community resources and benefits available for dementia patients can significantly ease financial burdens. Many organizations offer support services, grants, or programs specifically aimed at assisting those with early onset dementia and their families. It is beneficial to research local and national resources, including non-profits and government assistance programs, to determine eligibility and available support options. These resources can help cover costs related to care, therapy, and other necessary services, improving overall financial stability.

Technology can also play a vital role in managing finances. There are numerous applications and tools designed to simplify budgeting and expense tracking, making it easier for individuals with dementia and their caregivers to keep tabs on their financial situation. Using digital banking and automated payments can reduce the likelihood of missed bills and late fees, providing peace of mind. Additionally, many of these technologies offer reminders and alerts, which can be particularly helpful for those experiencing memory difficulties.

Finally, it is essential to have legal and financial plans in place to prepare for the future. Establishing advanced directives, wills, and powers of attorney ensures that an individual's wishes regarding healthcare and financial decisions are respected, even if they become unable to communicate those wishes themselves. Consulting with a legal professional who specializes in elder law or dementia-related issues can provide valuable guidance in this area. By taking proactive steps to manage finances and resources, individuals with early onset dementia can maintain greater control over their lives and ensure their needs are met.

Chapter 8: Staying Informed: Research and Clinical Trials

Current Research on Dementia

Current research on dementia is expanding our understanding of the condition, particularly as it affects individuals diagnosed at an earlier age. Researchers are exploring the biological mechanisms that lead to early onset dementia, focusing on genetic, environmental, and lifestyle factors that may contribute to its development. This research is crucial for identifying potential biomarkers that could lead to earlier diagnosis and more personalized treatment options. By understanding the underlying causes, scientists aim to create targeted therapies that could slow disease progression and improve quality of life for those affected.

Studies are also investigating the role of nutrition and diet in dementia prevention and management. Emerging evidence suggests that certain dietary patterns, such as the Mediterranean or DASH diets, may lower the risk of cognitive decline. Researchers are examining how specific nutrients, such as omega-3 fatty acids, antioxidants, and vitamins, impact brain health. This research is vital for patients and caregivers as it can inform dietary choices that may help maintain cognitive function and overall well-being. Engaging with nutritionists and dietitians who specialize in dementia care can further enhance these efforts.

Technology is another vibrant area of research aimed at supporting dementia patients and their caregivers. Innovations in assistive technologies, such as smart home devices, monitoring systems, and communication aids, are being developed to enhance independence and safety for individuals living with dementia. Studies are exploring the efficacy of these technologies in daily living, social engagement, and cognitive stimulation. These tools can empower patients, help manage symptoms, and provide peace of mind for caregivers, making it essential for patients to stay informed about available resources.

Clinical trials are a fundamental component of dementia research, providing insights into new treatments and interventions. Patients are encouraged to consider participating in these trials, as they may offer access to cutting-edge therapies not yet available to the general public. Current trials are investigating a range of options, from drug therapies targeting amyloid plaques to non-pharmacological interventions focused on cognitive rehabilitation. Participation in clinical trials not only contributes to the advancement of knowledge in dementia care but can also provide patients with valuable support and resources throughout the process.

Finally, research is increasingly recognizing the importance of mental health in the context of dementia. Studies are examining the psychological impact of an early onset dementia diagnosis on patients and their families. Addressing mental health through counseling, support groups, and alternative therapies is becoming a priority in holistic dementia care. This focus on mental well-being is essential for fostering resilience and coping strategies among patients and caregivers alike, ensuring that emotional support is an integral part of the journey with dementia. As research continues to evolve, staying connected with these developments can empower patients and caregivers to make informed decisions about their care.

How to Participate in Clinical Trials

Participating in clinical trials can offer valuable opportunities for individuals with early onset dementia and their caregivers. Clinical trials are research studies designed to test new treatments, medications, or interventions to determine their safety and effectiveness. By participating, you not only contribute to the advancement of medical knowledge but may also gain access to cutting-edge therapies that are not yet widely available. This can potentially improve your quality of life and provide you with new options for managing your condition.

To participate in a clinical trial, the first step is to find a suitable study. You can start by consulting with your healthcare provider, who can help identify ongoing trials that align with your specific condition and needs. Websites such as clinicaltrials.gov provide comprehensive databases of studies and their eligibility criteria. Look for trials that focus on early onset dementia and assess whether you meet the requirements. Each study will have specific inclusion and exclusion criteria based on age, symptom severity, and overall health.

Once you identify a potential trial, reach out to the research team for more information. They can provide details about the study's purpose, procedures, and what participation entails. It is essential to ask questions regarding the potential risks and benefits, the duration of the trial, and any required visits or assessments. Understanding these factors will help you make an informed decision about whether to participate. Involving your caregiver in this discussion can also provide additional support and clarity.

Before enrolling, you will be required to provide informed consent. This process ensures that you fully understand the study and agree to participate voluntarily. The research team will explain the trial's goals, procedures, and any potential risks involved. It is crucial to take your time during this stage, asking for clarifications on anything that is unclear. If you have concerns about your ability to comprehend the information due to cognitive challenges, request assistance from a trusted family member or caregiver.

Participating in a clinical trial can be a fulfilling experience, connecting you with a community of researchers and other individuals facing similar challenges. It may involve regular visits to the research site, where you can receive comprehensive care and support. Additionally, many trials offer compensation for your time and travel expenses. By contributing to research, you are not only advocating for your well-being but also paving the way for future advancements in the treatment of early onset dementia, ultimately benefiting others who may face similar circumstances.

Understanding New Treatments and Innovations

The landscape of dementia treatment is evolving rapidly, particularly with regard to early onset dementia. As researchers and healthcare providers deepen their understanding of the condition, new treatments and innovations are emerging that aim to improve the quality of life for patients. This subchapter focuses on the latest advancements in medical treatments, lifestyle approaches, and supportive technologies that can make a meaningful difference in managing the symptoms of early onset dementia. It is essential for patients and caregivers to stay informed about these developments, as they can play a pivotal role in enhancing daily life and fostering a sense of agency.

Pharmaceutical research is at the forefront of innovation in dementia care. Recently, several new medications have entered clinical trials, targeting specific symptoms and underlying mechanisms of the disease. These treatments range from cholinesterase inhibitors, which may help improve cognitive function, to novel therapies that aim to address amyloid plaques in the brain. Understanding these options and discussing them with healthcare providers can help patients and their families make informed decisions about potential therapies, tailoring approaches to individual needs and preferences.

In addition to pharmacological advancements, lifestyle modifications are increasingly recognized for their impact on dementia management. Innovations in nutrition and diet have shown promise in supporting cognitive health. Diets rich in antioxidants, omega-3 fatty acids, and vitamins can potentially slow cognitive decline. Programs that promote physical activity and social engagement also contribute to overall well-being, emphasizing the importance of maintaining an active lifestyle. Caregivers play a crucial role in facilitating these lifestyle changes, ensuring that patients have access to healthy foods and opportunities for social interaction.

Technology is revolutionizing the way individuals with early onset dementia engage with their environment. Smart home devices, wearable technology, and mobile applications are designed to assist in day-to-day activities, offering reminders for medication and appointments, as well as providing cognitive stimulation through games and exercises. These tools not only help patients maintain independence but also serve as valuable resources for caregivers, allowing them to monitor health and safety more effectively. Embracing these technologies can significantly enhance the living experience for both patients and their support networks.

Lastly, ongoing research and clinical trials play a critical role in the fight against dementia. Participation in clinical trials can provide access to cutting-edge treatments and therapeutic approaches that are not yet widely available. Additionally, understanding the ethical and legal implications of these trials is important for patients and their families. Engaging with research initiatives not only contributes to personal health but also advances the broader understanding of dementia, potentially leading to breakthroughs that can benefit future generations. By remaining informed and proactive, patients and caregivers can navigate the complexities of early onset dementia with greater confidence and support.

Chapter 9: Mental Health and Well-being

Addressing Emotional Health

Addressing emotional health is a crucial aspect of living well with early onset dementia. Emotional well-being significantly influences overall quality of life, and individuals with dementia may experience a range of emotions, including sadness, frustration, and anxiety. Recognizing these feelings and understanding their impact can empower patients and caregivers to seek appropriate support and strategies. Acknowledging emotional health is not only vital for patients but also for caregivers, who often face their own emotional challenges while providing care.

Engaging in open communication about feelings can help both patients and caregivers navigate the emotional landscape of dementia. Creating a safe space for discussions encourages honesty and fosters understanding. Patients should feel comfortable expressing their fears and frustrations, while caregivers can share their concerns and experiences. This mutual exchange can strengthen relationships and enhance emotional support. Utilizing tools such as journals or art therapy can also facilitate expression, allowing patients to articulate their feelings in creative ways that may be more comfortable than traditional conversation.

In addition to communication, emotional health can be supported through structured activities that promote engagement and positivity. Participating in dementia-friendly activities—such as music therapy, gardening, or simple crafts—can stimulate the brain and uplift mood. These activities not only provide enjoyment but also foster a sense of accomplishment and purpose. Caregivers are encouraged to explore various options and identify what resonates most with the individual, tailoring activities to their preferences and capabilities.

Nutrition also plays a vital role in emotional health, as certain foods can impact mood and cognitive function. A balanced diet that includes fruits, vegetables, whole grains, and healthy fats can support brain health and, consequently, emotional well-being. Caregivers can assist patients in making dietary choices that promote emotional stability, incorporating foods rich in omega-3 fatty acids, antioxidants, and vitamins. Meal planning together can also serve as a bonding activity, reinforcing social connections and providing a sense of routine.

Finally, addressing emotional health requires awareness of available resources and support systems. Mental health professionals, support groups, and educational materials can provide invaluable assistance. Caregivers should not hesitate to seek help when needed, as their emotional health is equally important. By prioritizing emotional well-being for both patients and caregivers, the challenges of early onset dementia can be managed more effectively, leading to a more fulfilling and connected life.

Coping Strategies for Stress and Anxiety

Coping with stress and anxiety is crucial for individuals living with early onset dementia, as these feelings can exacerbate cognitive decline and negatively affect overall quality of life. It is essential to recognize the signs of stress and anxiety, which may include increased agitation, changes in sleep patterns, or withdrawal from social activities. By identifying these symptoms early, patients and caregivers can implement effective coping strategies to manage these feelings. Understanding that anxiety is a common response to the uncertainties associated with dementia can help normalize these feelings and encourage proactive management.

One effective coping strategy is the establishment of a structured daily routine. Predictability can provide comfort and reduce anxiety, as individuals with early onset dementia often feel overwhelmed by changes and unexpected events. A consistent schedule that includes regular meal times, exercise, and leisure activities can create a sense of stability. Caregivers can help by outlining daily plans and engaging patients in the process, fostering a sense of control and involvement. Additionally, incorporating relaxation techniques, such as deep breathing exercises or mindfulness meditation, can further alleviate stress and promote a sense of calm.

Engaging in dementia-friendly activities is another valuable strategy for managing stress and anxiety. Activities that are enjoyable and stimulating can distract from negative thoughts and provide opportunities for social interaction. Creative pursuits such as painting, music, or gardening can evoke positive emotions and enhance cognitive engagement. Caregivers can facilitate these activities by focusing on the patient's interests and abilities, ensuring that the experience remains enjoyable rather than overwhelming. Group activities, such as support groups or community events tailored for those with dementia, can also foster connection and reduce feelings of isolation.

Nutrition plays a significant role in emotional well-being and cognitive health. A balanced diet rich in antioxidants, omega-3 fatty acids, and vitamins can support brain function and help manage mood. Caregivers should work with healthcare professionals to develop meal plans that are not only nutritious but also cater to the patient's tastes and preferences. Encouraging healthy eating habits can create a sense of routine and normalcy, which is beneficial for emotional stability. Additionally, staying hydrated and limiting caffeine and sugar can further contribute to improved mental health.

Technology aids offer innovative solutions for coping with stress and anxiety among dementia patients. Mobile apps designed for relaxation, mood tracking, and cognitive exercises can provide both entertainment and mental stimulation. Virtual reality experiences can immerse patients in calming environments, helping to reduce anxiety levels. Caregivers can assist with navigating these technologies, ensuring that patients feel comfortable and confident in their use. By integrating technology into daily life, patients can access additional resources for managing stress while maintaining their independence and engagement.

Seeking Professional Support

Seeking professional support is a crucial step for individuals living with early onset dementia and their caregivers. As the progression of dementia can vary significantly from person to person, professional guidance can help tailor strategies to individual needs. Healthcare professionals, including neurologists, geriatricians, and neuropsychologists, can provide comprehensive assessments, which are essential for accurate diagnosis and treatment planning. These assessments not only clarify the type of dementia but also help identify additional health concerns that may impact overall well-being.

In addition to medical professionals, seeking support from mental health experts is vital. Early onset dementia can lead to feelings of anxiety, depression, and isolation. Psychologists and counselors specializing in dementia care can offer therapeutic interventions that focus on coping strategies, emotional support, and enhancing quality of life. They can also assist caregivers in managing their own emotional health, which is crucial as they navigate the challenges of supporting a loved one with dementia.

Engaging with support groups can also be beneficial. These groups provide a platform for individuals with early onset dementia and their families to share experiences, advice, and resources. Connecting with others facing similar challenges can foster a sense of community and understanding. Many organizations offer structured programs that include educational workshops, social activities, and access to informative resources that can empower patients and caregivers alike.

Exploring technology aids can enhance daily living and communication for individuals with dementia. Professionals can recommend various tools, from reminder apps to devices that facilitate social interaction. These technologies can assist with memory recall, scheduling, and even safety monitoring, allowing individuals to maintain a level of independence while ensuring they remain connected with their support networks. Familiarizing oneself with these tools under professional guidance can significantly improve both daily functioning and overall quality of life.

Lastly, legal and financial planning is an essential aspect of managing early onset dementia. Consulting with legal professionals who specialize in elder law can help individuals and their families navigate complex decisions regarding power of attorney, healthcare directives, and financial management. Being proactive in these areas can alleviate stress and uncertainty, allowing individuals to focus on living well. Engaging with professionals in these fields ensures that both patients and caregivers are equipped with the necessary tools and knowledge to make informed decisions as they adapt to the realities of dementia.

Chapter 10: Communication Strategies

Effective Communication Techniques

Effective communication techniques are essential for maintaining connections and ensuring that individuals with early onset dementia can express their needs and feelings. One effective approach is to simplify language and use straightforward words. Avoiding complex sentences and jargon can help reduce confusion. When engaging in conversation, it is beneficial to speak slowly and clearly, allowing the listener time to process the information. Additionally, using non-verbal cues such as gestures, facial expressions, and eye contact can enhance understanding and reinforce the spoken message.

Active listening is another crucial technique that can significantly improve communication. Caregivers and family members should focus on being present during conversations, minimizing distractions, and giving their full attention. This can involve nodding in acknowledgment and providing verbal affirmations like "I see" or "Go on." By demonstrating that they are genuinely interested and engaged, caregivers can encourage patients to share their thoughts and feelings more openly, fostering a supportive environment for dialogue.

Using visual aids can also be beneficial in enhancing communication with individuals living with early onset dementia. Pictures, written cues, or visual schedules can help clarify messages and provide context for conversations. For example, showing a photograph of a loved one while discussing them can create a more tangible connection. Visual aids not only assist with memory recall but also reduce anxiety, as patients can refer to these resources if they struggle to understand or remember information.

Establishing a routine can serve as a foundation for effective communication. Predictable schedules allow patients to become familiar with daily activities and interactions, reducing stress and confusion. Consistency in communication practices, such as using the same phrases or prompts for common activities, can also help reinforce understanding. Caregivers should be patient and flexible, adapting their communication style as needed, while remaining supportive and encouraging.

Lastly, encouraging the use of technology can facilitate communication for those living with early onset dementia. Many tools, such as tablets or smartphones, come equipped with applications designed to support memory and communication. Video calls can help maintain social connections with family and friends, combating feelings of isolation. Caregivers should explore various technological aids that align with the patient's preferences and comfort level, ensuring that these tools enhance rather than complicate their communication experience. By integrating these effective communication techniques, individuals with early onset dementia can feel more empowered and connected, fostering a greater sense of well-being.

Non-Verbal Communication

Non-verbal communication plays a crucial role in how individuals express their thoughts and feelings, especially for those living with early onset dementia. As cognitive abilities decline, verbal communication may become more challenging, making non-verbal cues an essential tool for conveying emotions and intentions. Understanding and utilizing non-verbal communication can enhance interactions with loved ones, caregivers, and healthcare providers, fostering a more supportive and compassionate environment.

Body language, facial expressions, and gestures are key components of non-verbal communication. These signals can express a wide range of emotions such as joy, sadness, frustration, or confusion without the need for words. For individuals with early onset dementia, paying attention to these cues can provide valuable insights into their emotional state and needs. Caregivers and family members can benefit from being observant of changes in posture, eye contact, and facial expressions, as these non-verbal signals can indicate whether someone is comfortable, agitated, or in need of assistance.

Another important aspect of non-verbal communication is the use of touch. A gentle hug, a reassuring hand on the shoulder, or simply holding hands can convey support and understanding. Touch can often bridge the gap when words fail, providing comfort and connection. It is important for caregivers to be sensitive to the preferences of individuals with dementia regarding touch, as it can be a source of comfort for some while causing distress for others. Establishing a trusting relationship with appropriate non-verbal cues can significantly enhance the emotional well-being of individuals with early onset dementia.

Visual aids and symbols can also facilitate non-verbal communication. Pictures, gestures, and visual prompts can help convey messages more clearly. For example, using a communication board with images representing common needs or feelings can aid in expressing thoughts without relying solely on verbal skills. Caregivers can create simple visual schedules or reminders that help individuals with dementia understand daily activities, thereby reducing anxiety and confusion. Engaging in activities that incorporate visual elements, such as art or music therapy, can also encourage non-verbal expression and communication.

Lastly, creating a calm and positive environment can enhance non-verbal communication. Reducing background noise, ensuring good lighting, and eliminating distractions can help individuals focus on non-verbal cues, both from themselves and others. Encouraging a relaxed atmosphere allows for more effective communication, as it enables individuals to feel safe and understood. By fostering an environment that prioritizes non-verbal communication, caregivers and family members can help individuals with early onset dementia navigate their experiences and enhance their quality of life.

Engaging Conversations

Engaging conversations play a crucial role in maintaining the well-being and quality of life for individuals living with early onset dementia. Communication can become challenging as the disease progresses, but it is essential to create opportunities for meaningful interactions. Engaging conversations can stimulate the mind, evoke memories, and foster connections with caregivers and loved ones. By focusing on shared interests, past experiences, and current feelings, individuals with early onset dementia can experience a sense of belonging and purpose.

To facilitate engaging conversations, it is beneficial to create a comfortable and supportive environment. This involves minimizing distractions and ensuring that the surroundings are calm and quiet. Caregivers and family members should approach conversations with patience and understanding. Using clear, simple language while allowing ample time for the individual to respond can enhance understanding and reduce frustration. Active listening is vital; showing genuine interest in the responses encourages individuals to share their thoughts and feelings more freely.

Incorporating familiar topics can also enhance engagement. Discussing hobbies, favorite books, music, or family stories can spark joyful memories and encourage participation in the conversation. Utilizing visual aids, such as photographs or meaningful objects, can help trigger memories and promote discussion. Additionally, caregivers might consider asking open-ended questions that invite elaboration rather than simple yes or no answers, fostering a richer dialogue and deeper connection.

Technology can serve as an excellent tool for enhancing conversations. Video calls with family members or friends who live far away can help maintain relationships and provide emotional support. There are also applications designed to promote cognitive engagement through games and storytelling, making interactions more enjoyable and stimulating. Incorporating these tools into daily routines can help individuals with early onset dementia stay connected and engaged with their loved ones.

Ultimately, engaging conversations are about connection, understanding, and support. They can significantly enhance the quality of life for individuals living with early onset dementia by providing opportunities for expression and interaction. By creating a nurturing environment, using familiar topics, and embracing technology, caregivers and loved ones can facilitate meaningful conversations that enrich the lives of those affected by dementia.

Chapter 11: Alternative Therapies for Dementia Management

Overview of Alternative Therapies

Alternative therapies encompass a variety of non-conventional approaches that can complement traditional medical treatments for early onset dementia. These therapies often focus on holistic well-being, addressing not only cognitive function but also emotional, physical, and social aspects of health. By providing additional support, alternative therapies can enhance the quality of life for individuals living with dementia, helping them maintain independence and dignity as they navigate their condition.

One of the most commonly explored alternative therapies is music therapy. This approach utilizes music to promote cognitive stimulation and emotional connection, often leading to improvements in mood and social interaction. Research has shown that familiar tunes can evoke memories and emotions, allowing individuals with early onset dementia to engage with their past in meaningful ways. Caregivers can also benefit from music therapy, as it fosters shared experiences and can create a calming environment during challenging moments.

Art therapy is another valuable alternative therapy that encourages self-expression and creativity. Through various artistic mediums, individuals can communicate feelings and thoughts that may be difficult to articulate verbally. This form of therapy not only aids in cognitive engagement but also promotes relaxation and reduces anxiety. Engaging in art can provide a sense of accomplishment and joy, which is vital for emotional health in dementia patients. Caregivers can facilitate these sessions, fostering a supportive atmosphere that encourages creativity.

Mindfulness and meditation practices offer additional benefits for those living with early onset dementia. These techniques help individuals focus on the present moment, reducing stress and anxiety associated with cognitive decline. Mindfulness has been shown to enhance overall mental well-being and may even improve cognitive functions such as attention and memory. Caregivers can participate in mindfulness exercises alongside their loved ones, creating a shared experience that strengthens their bond and encourages emotional resilience.

Lastly, integrating nutrition as an alternative therapy can play a crucial role in managing dementia symptoms. A balanced diet rich in antioxidants, omega-3 fatty acids, and other vital nutrients supports brain health and may slow cognitive decline. Caregivers should focus on providing meals that are not only nutritious but also enjoyable, as mealtime can be an opportunity for social engagement. By combining nutrition with other alternative therapies, individuals with early onset dementia can benefit from a comprehensive approach to their care, enhancing both their physical and mental well-being.

Mindfulness and Meditation

Mindfulness and meditation have emerged as valuable tools for individuals living with early onset dementia. These practices focus on fostering a state of awareness and presence, helping patients navigate the challenges associated with cognitive decline. By encouraging individuals to engage in the present moment, mindfulness and meditation can alleviate stress and anxiety, which are common among those facing dementia. Incorporating these practices into daily routines may enhance overall well-being and improve emotional health.

Mindfulness involves paying attention to one's thoughts, feelings, and sensations without judgment. For dementia patients, this practice can help in managing feelings of frustration or confusion that often arise from memory loss and cognitive impairment. Simple techniques such as mindful breathing or body scans can be effective. For instance, spending a few moments observing the breath can create a sense of calm and grounding, allowing individuals to refocus their thoughts and emotions. Caregivers can facilitate this process by guiding patients through mindfulness exercises, fostering a supportive environment that promotes relaxation and connection.

Meditation, on the other hand, offers a structured approach to mindfulness. Various forms of meditation, such as guided imagery or loving-kindness meditation, can be particularly beneficial. These techniques involve visualizing positive experiences or sending thoughts of compassion to oneself and others. Such practices can help dementia patients cultivate a sense of peace and acceptance, reducing feelings of isolation and distress. Engaging in meditation with a caregiver or in a group setting can also enhance social interaction, creating a community support system that is vital for emotional health.

Establishing a regular mindfulness or meditation practice may seem daunting, but it can be easily integrated into daily life. Patients can start with just a few minutes each day, gradually increasing the duration as they become more comfortable. Caregivers play a crucial role in this process by providing encouragement and joining in the practice. Together, they can create a routine that includes mindfulness exercises, such as mindful walking in nature or sitting in a quiet space, which can significantly improve mood and cognitive function.

In conclusion, mindfulness and meditation offer promising avenues for improving the quality of life for individuals with early onset dementia. These practices not only help in managing emotional challenges but also foster a sense of community and support through shared experiences. By embracing mindfulness and meditation, patients and their caregivers can create a more enriching daily life, promoting better mental health and emotional resilience as they navigate the complexities of dementia.

Art and Music Therapy

Art and music therapy have emerged as powerful tools in the management of early onset dementia, offering patients unique ways to express themselves and engage with the world around them. These therapies harness the inherent creativity in individuals, allowing them to connect with their emotions, memories, and even their identities. For patients, engaging in art and music can provide a sense of purpose and achievement, which may help alleviate feelings of frustration or isolation that often accompany dementia.

Art therapy involves the use of various artistic mediums, such as painting, drawing, and sculpture, to facilitate communication and self-expression. This form of therapy does not require prior artistic skills; rather, it focuses on the process of creation rather than the final product. Patients can explore their thoughts and feelings through visual art, which can lead to improved mood and cognitive function. Caregivers can support this activity by providing a variety of materials and creating a comfortable space for artistic exploration.

Music therapy, similarly, utilizes the power of sound and rhythm to promote emotional well-being and cognitive engagement. Listening to familiar songs or participating in music-making activities can evoke memories and stimulate brain function. Music has a unique ability to transcend language barriers and may help patients communicate more effectively, even when verbal skills decline. Caregivers can enhance this experience by curating playlists of songs that hold personal significance to the patient, fostering a sense of nostalgia and connection.

Both art and music therapies offer dementia patients opportunities for social interaction, which is crucial for mental health. Group sessions can create a sense of community and belonging, reducing feelings of loneliness. Participating in these therapeutic activities alongside others can encourage patients to share their experiences, fostering relationships and support networks. Caregivers play a vital role in facilitating these group sessions, ensuring that the environment is inclusive and encouraging for all participants.

Incorporating art and music therapy into the daily routine can lead to lasting benefits for those living with early onset dementia. These activities not only promote cognitive engagement but also enhance emotional well-being by providing an outlet for expression and connection. As caregivers and loved ones, it is essential to recognize and encourage these forms of therapy, as they can significantly improve the quality of life for dementia patients. By embracing the creative arts, patients can rediscover joy, build resilience, and maintain a meaningful connection to their surroundings.

Chapter 12: Looking Ahead: Planning for the Future

Setting Goals for Living Well

Setting goals for living well with early onset dementia is an essential aspect of maintaining quality of life. Goals provide a sense of purpose and direction, which can be particularly beneficial for individuals facing the challenges of dementia. By establishing clear, achievable objectives, patients can foster a greater sense of control over their circumstances. It is important to approach goal-setting with flexibility, recognizing that needs and capabilities may change over time. Engaging in this process can empower patients to focus on what they still enjoy and value in life.

One effective strategy for goal-setting is to employ the SMART criteria, ensuring that goals are Specific, Measurable, Achievable, Relevant, and Time-bound. For instance, rather than stating a vague goal such as "stay active," a SMART goal might be "participate in a 30-minute walk three times a week." This approach helps to clarify intentions and provides a framework for evaluating progress. Setting small, incremental goals can also foster motivation and provide opportunities for celebrating achievements, no matter how minor they may seem.

In addition to physical activity, it is vital to consider social engagement as part of the goal-setting process. Maintaining connections with family, friends, and support groups can significantly enhance emotional well-being. Goals such as attending a weekly support group meeting or scheduling regular phone calls with loved ones can help combat feelings of isolation. Caregivers can play a crucial role in this aspect by facilitating these interactions and encouraging patients to engage in community activities that interest them.

Nutrition and diet also play a critical role in living well with dementia. Setting dietary goals can help individuals focus on maintaining a balanced and healthy diet, which has been associated with cognitive health. Patients might aim to incorporate more fruits and vegetables into their meals or to reduce processed foods. Caregivers can assist by planning meals together, exploring new recipes, or even involving patients in grocery shopping, thereby enhancing their sense of autonomy and participation.

Finally, it is essential to recognize the importance of mental health in the goal-setting process. Goals related to mental wellness, such as practicing mindfulness or engaging in creative activities, can contribute significantly to emotional stability. Technology aids, such as apps designed for meditation or cognitive exercises, can be valuable resources in this regard. By setting goals that encompass physical, social, nutritional, and mental aspects of life, individuals with early onset dementia can create a comprehensive framework for living well, fostering resilience and a positive outlook amidst their diagnosis.

Adapting to Changes in Health

Adapting to changes in health is an essential aspect of managing early onset dementia. As the condition progresses, individuals may experience a range of cognitive and physical changes that can impact daily life. Recognizing and understanding these changes can help patients and their caregivers develop effective strategies to maintain quality of life. It is crucial to approach these adaptations with a proactive mindset, focusing on what can be controlled and improved rather than what is lost.

One of the first steps in adapting to health changes is to establish a routine that accommodates new abilities and challenges. Consistency can provide a sense of stability and security, which is particularly important for individuals with dementia. This routine might include daily activities that engage the mind and body, such as walking, puzzles, or art projects, which not only stimulate cognitive function but also enhance emotional well-being. Caregivers play a vital role in this process by helping to create an environment that is both supportive and adaptable, allowing for flexibility as needs evolve.

Nutrition and diet also play a significant role in health adaptation. Research suggests that certain diets, such as the Mediterranean diet, may have protective effects on cognitive function. Patients should focus on incorporating nutrient-rich foods, such as fruits, vegetables, whole grains, and healthy fats, into their meals. Caregivers can assist by planning and preparing meals that meet these dietary guidelines, making mealtime an opportunity for social interaction and engagement. Additionally, staying hydrated is crucial, as dehydration can exacerbate cognitive decline.

In today's digital age, technology offers numerous tools to assist individuals with early onset dementia. From reminder apps to wearable devices that track health metrics, these resources can help patients manage their daily activities more effectively. Caregivers should explore various technological aids that can enhance communication, safety, and independence. Training sessions on how to use these technologies can empower both patients and caregivers, fostering a sense of control over the condition.

Finally, emotional and mental health should be prioritized as part of the adaptation process. Open communication between patients and caregivers is vital for addressing feelings of frustration, anxiety, or sadness that may arise from health changes. Engaging in alternative therapies, such as mindfulness, music therapy, or art therapy, can provide additional emotional support and enhance cognitive engagement. Understanding that adapting to changes is a journey that requires patience and resilience can empower both patients and caregivers to navigate the complexities of early onset dementia together, focusing on living well despite the challenges.

Maintaining Hope and Resilience

Maintaining hope and resilience is crucial for individuals living with early onset dementia. As you navigate the challenges presented by this condition, fostering a mindset of hope can significantly impact your emotional well-being and overall quality of life. This subchapter explores practical strategies to cultivate hope, resilience, and a positive outlook, ensuring that you can adapt to the changes brought on by dementia while continuing to engage meaningfully with the world around you.

One of the key components of maintaining hope is setting realistic goals. Establishing small, achievable objectives can provide a sense of direction and purpose, which is essential for emotional health. For instance, consider setting daily or weekly goals related to hobbies or social interactions. Engaging in dementia-friendly activities such as art classes, music therapy, or storytelling can not only enhance your mood but also foster connections with others who understand your journey. These activities serve as a reminder that enjoyment and fulfillment are still attainable, even in the face of cognitive challenges.

Support networks are invaluable in promoting resilience. Staying connected with family, friends, and support groups can provide emotional sustenance and practical assistance. Sharing experiences with others who are also navigating the complexities of early onset dementia can create a sense of belonging and understanding. Caregivers can play a vital role in this process by encouraging open communication and actively participating in activities that promote social engagement. Together, you and your support network can create an environment where hope thrives and resilience is nurtured.

Nutrition and diet also play a significant role in maintaining cognitive health and emotional resilience. A balanced diet rich in fruits, vegetables, whole grains, and healthy fats can positively influence brain function. Consider exploring meal planning with your caregiver or family members to incorporate foods that support cognitive health while also being enjoyable. Additionally, engaging in cooking activities can serve as a therapeutic and social experience, allowing you to connect with loved ones while maintaining your independence in the kitchen.

Finally, embracing technology can enhance hope and resilience by providing tools for communication and engagement. There are various applications and devices designed specifically for individuals with dementia that can assist with memory, scheduling, and daily tasks. By utilizing these aids, you can maintain autonomy and stay connected with your loved ones, helping to mitigate feelings of isolation and frustration. Furthermore, participating in clinical trials or research studies can foster a sense of contribution to the broader understanding of dementia, instilling hope that progress is being made and that new treatments may emerge in the future.